IF YOU GIVE A CANC COLORING B(THEY WILL GET 10 MORE. BUT NONE AS AWESOME AS THIS ONE!

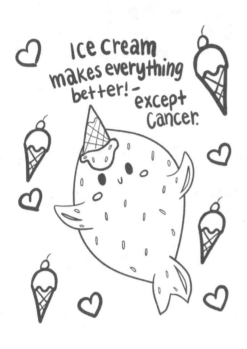

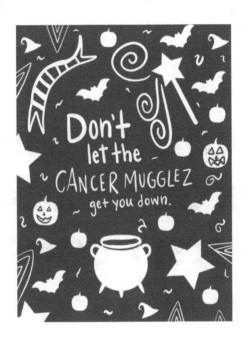

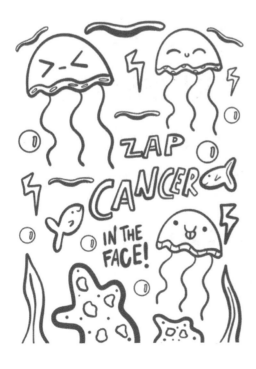

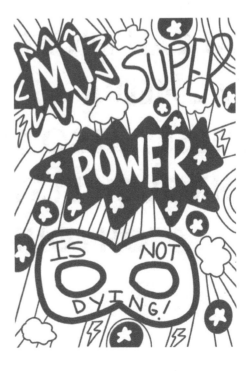

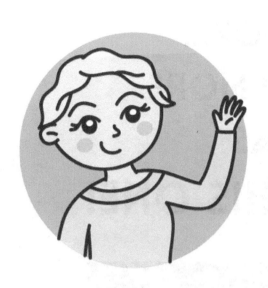

ohyoure sotough

ALL COLORING PAGES IN THIS BOOK ARE ORIGINAL WORKS OF ART BY CHELSEY GOMEZ AKA THE ARTIST KNOWN AS "OHYOURESOTOUGH"

YOU CAN FIND CHELSEY ACROSS ALL SOCIAL MEDIA AS "OHYOURESOTOUGH". CHELSEY ALSO SELLS HER ARTWORK THROUGH ETSY UNDER THE NAME "OHYOURESOTOUGH"

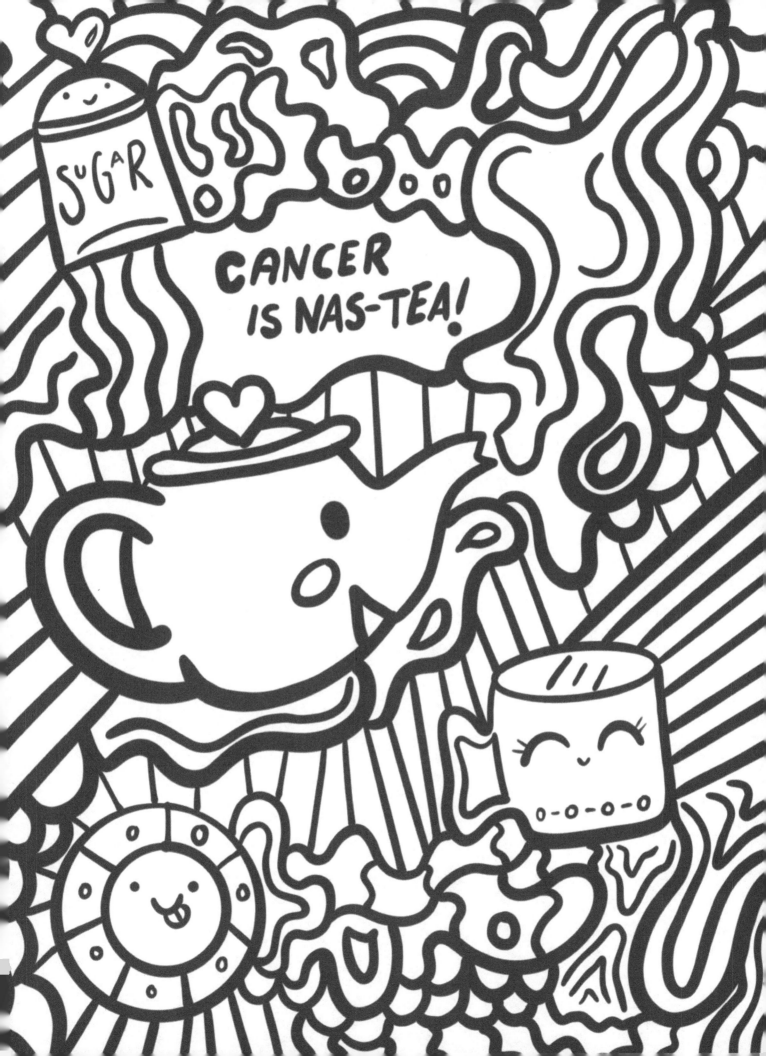

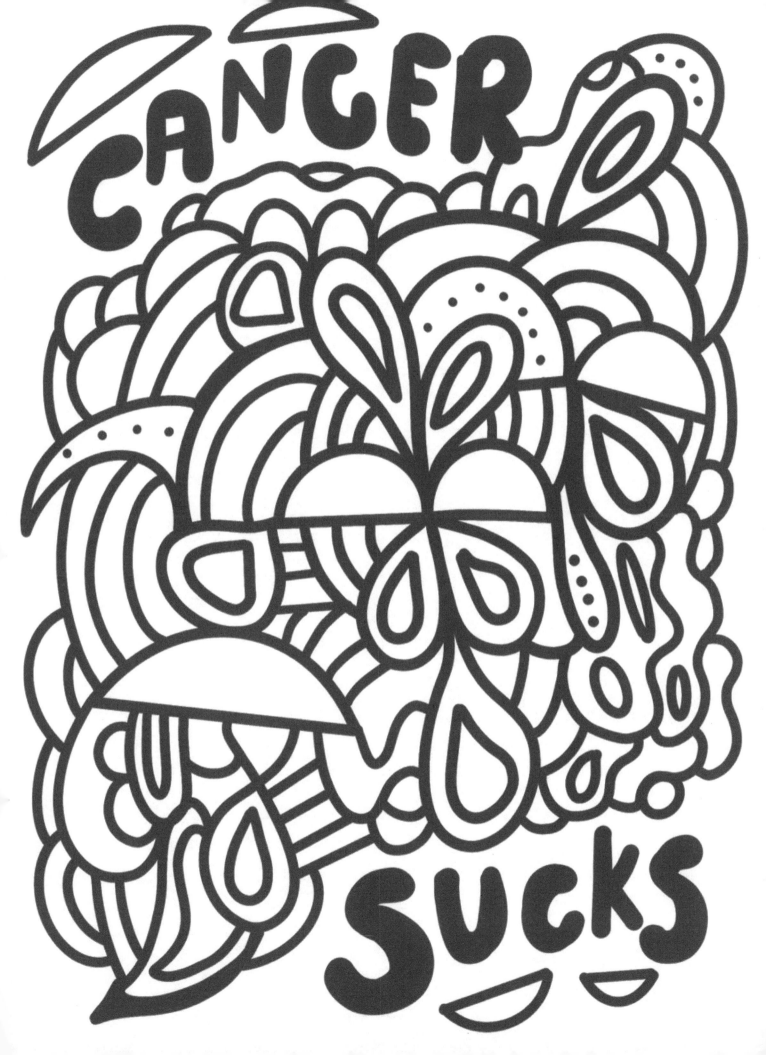

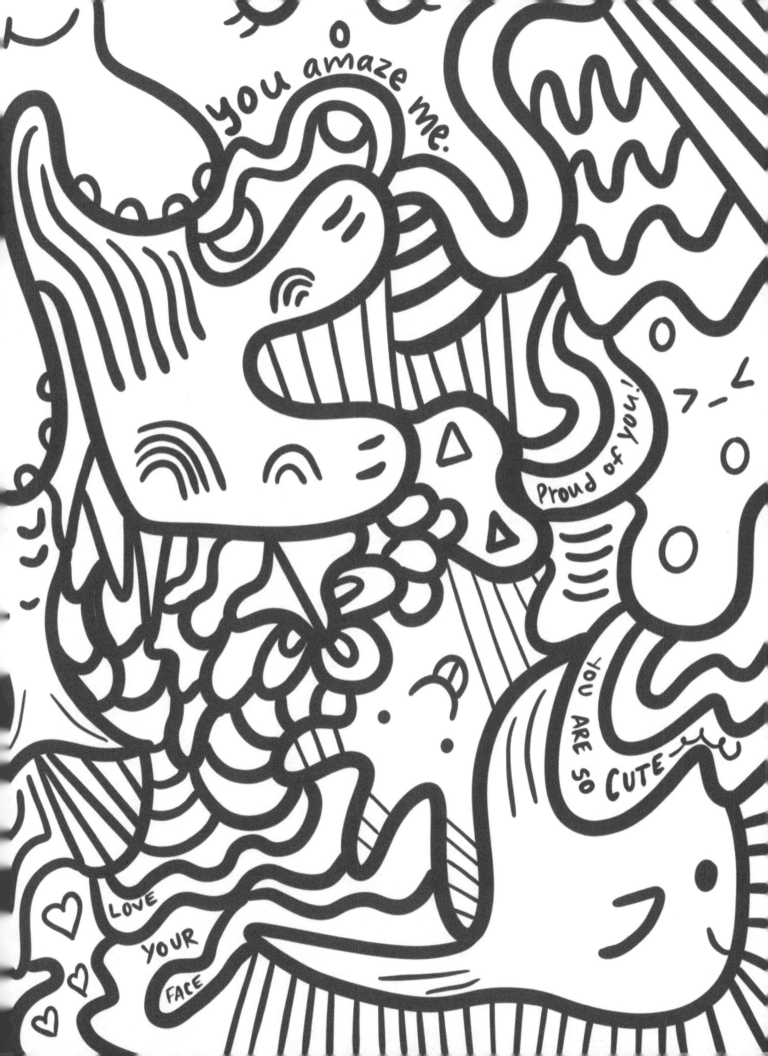

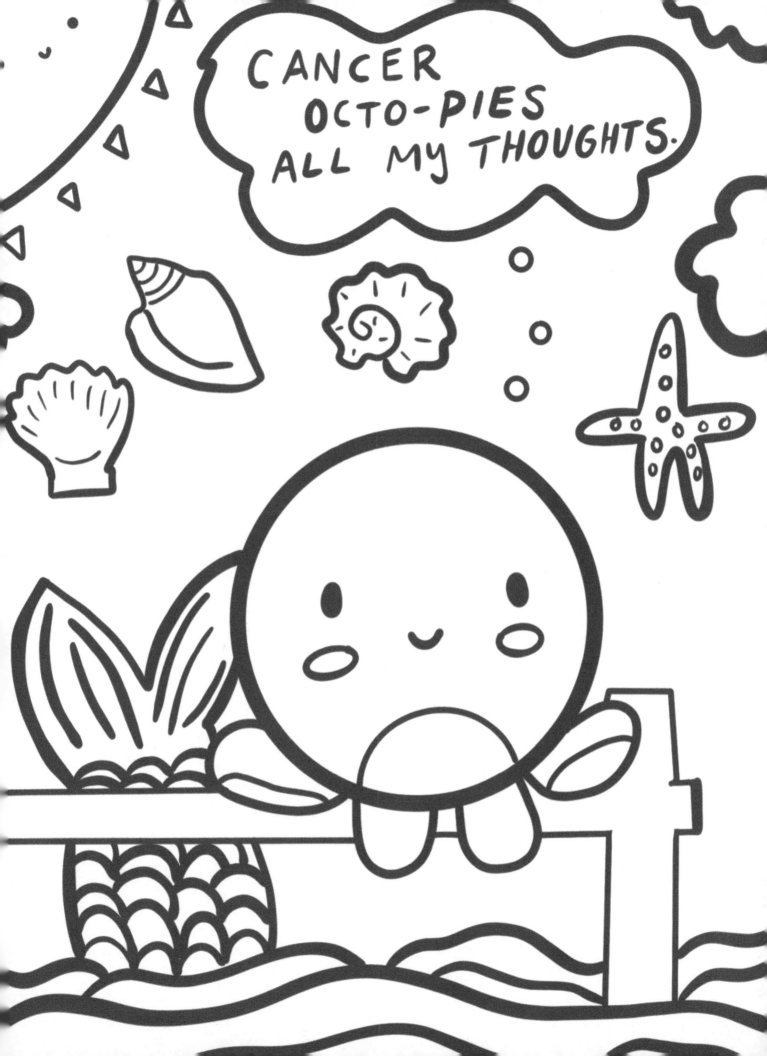

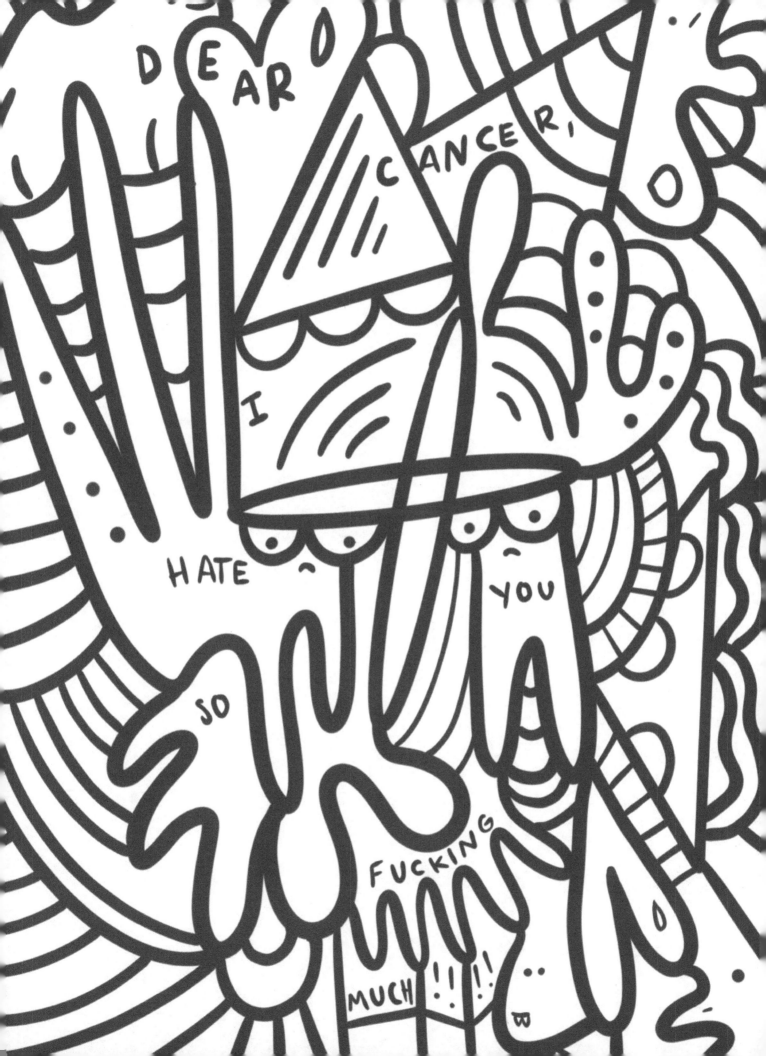

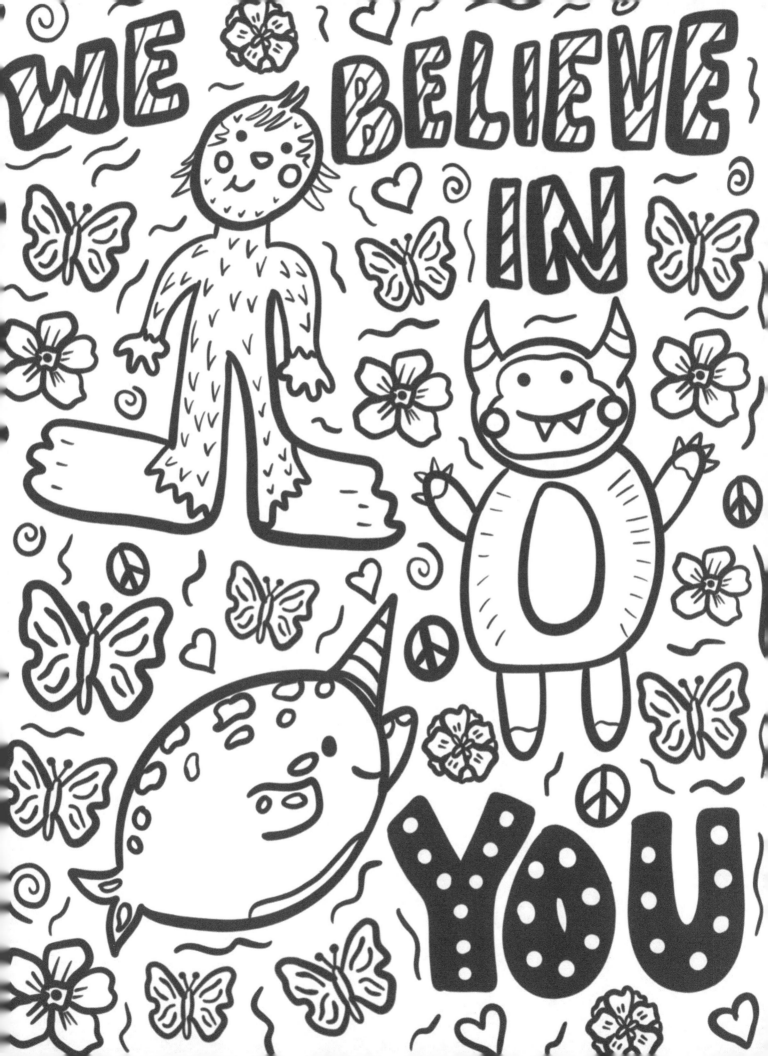

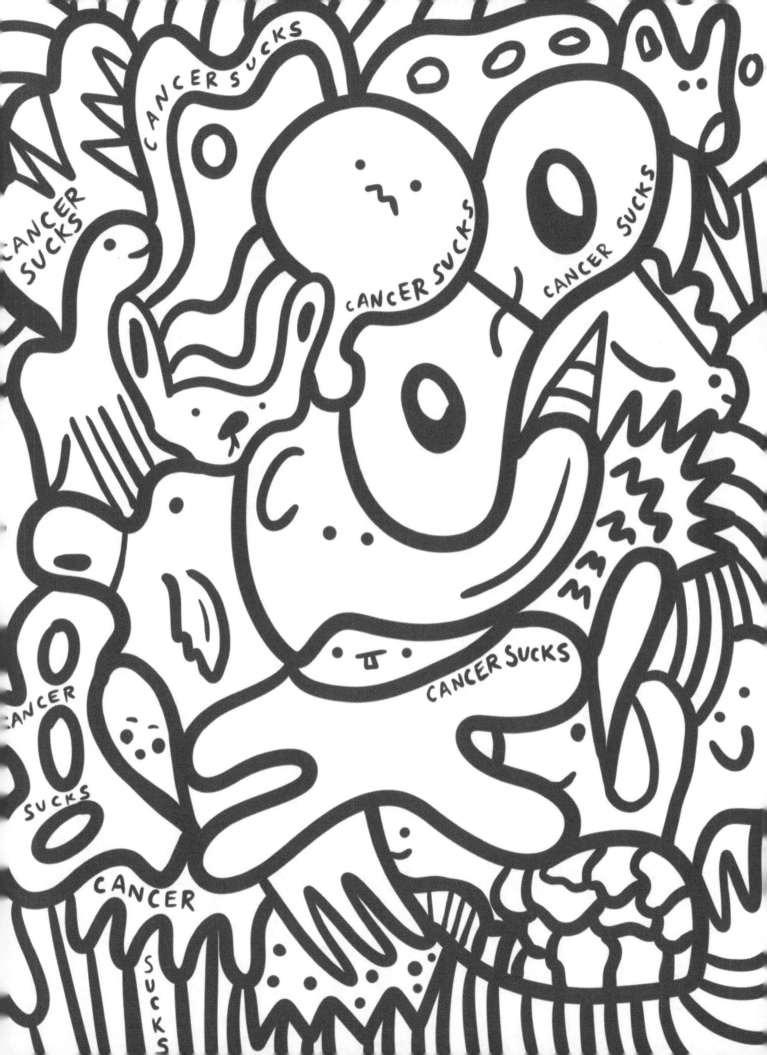

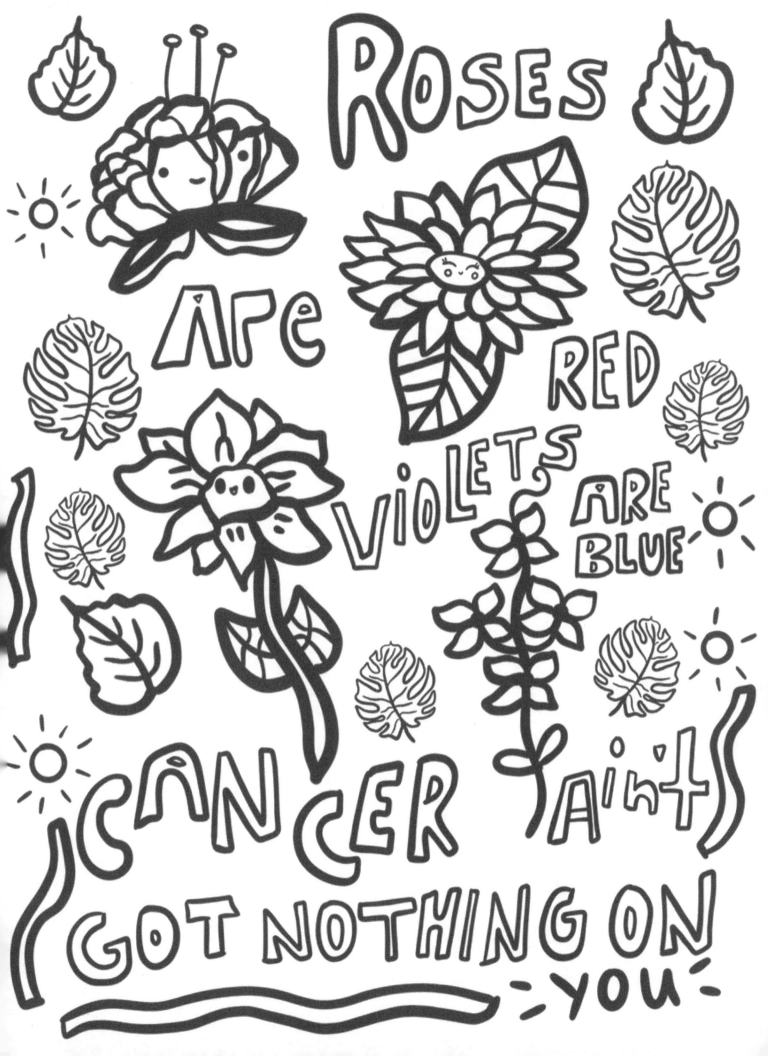

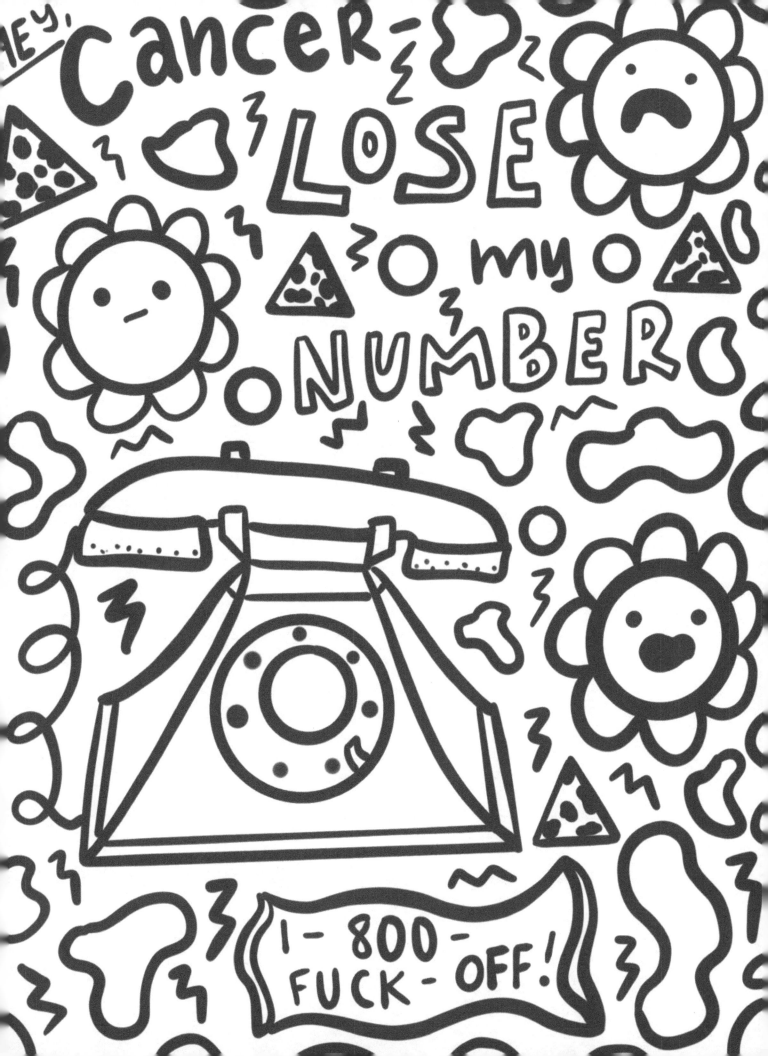

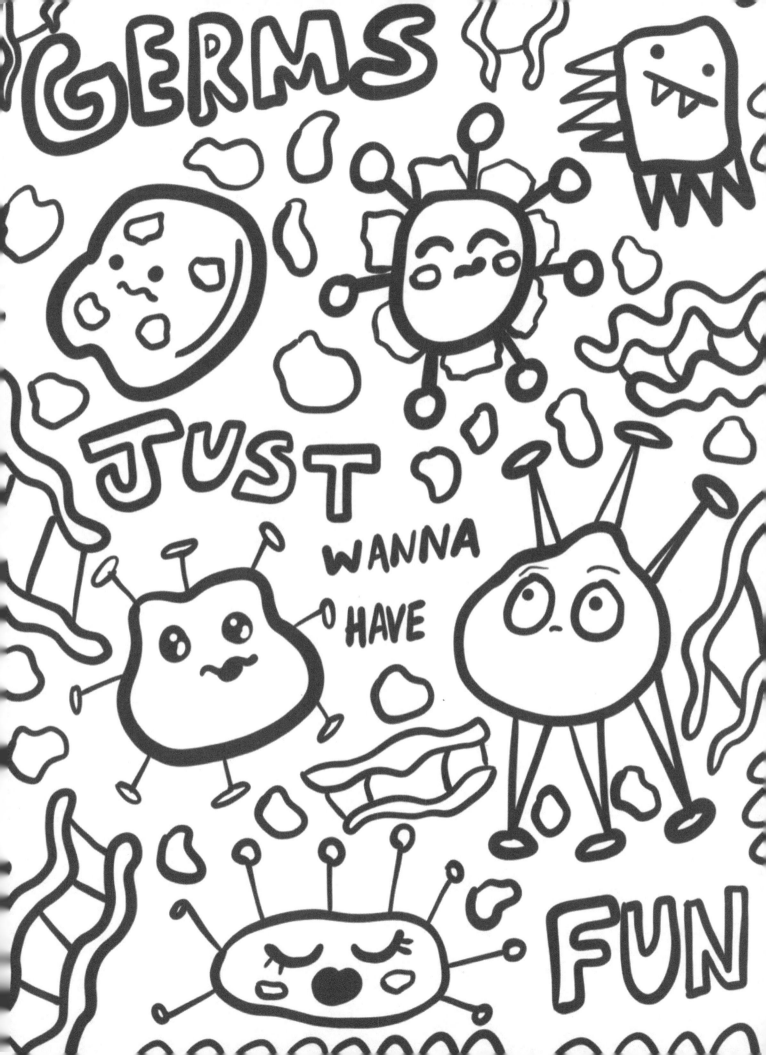

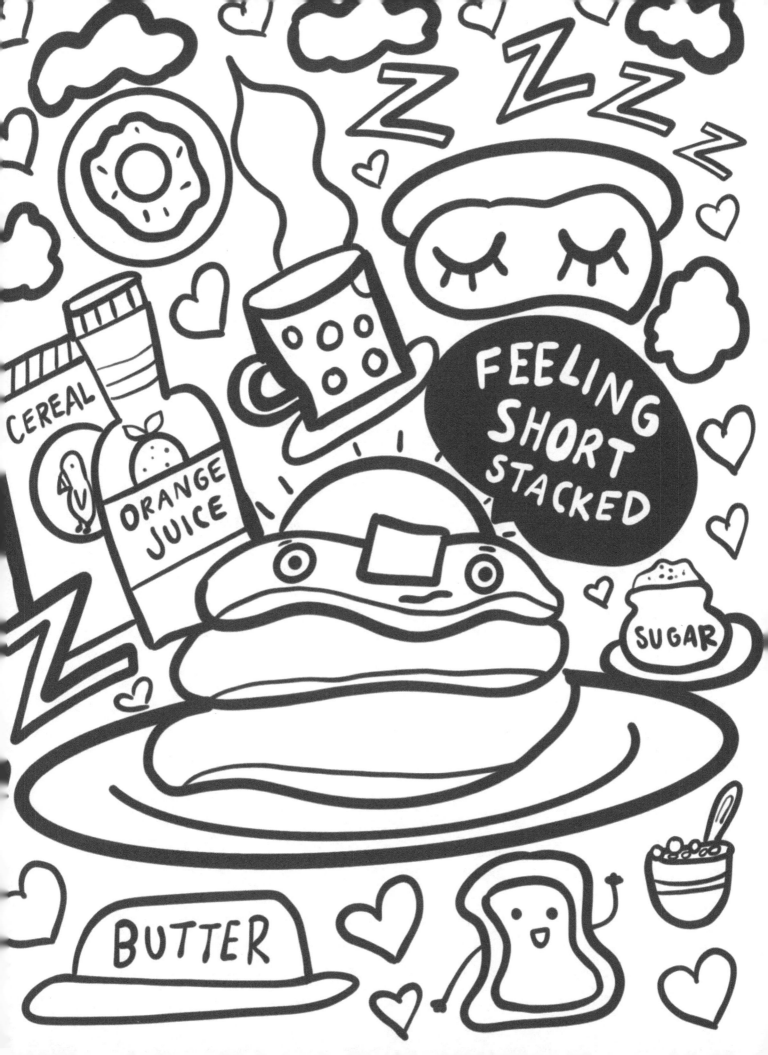

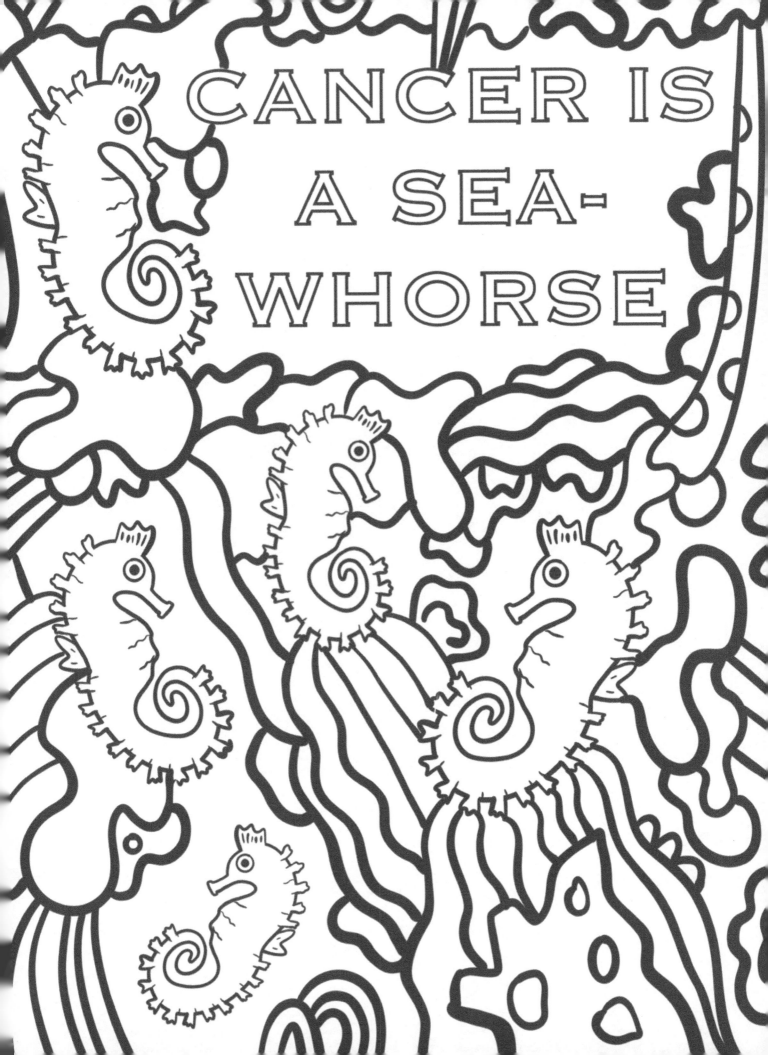

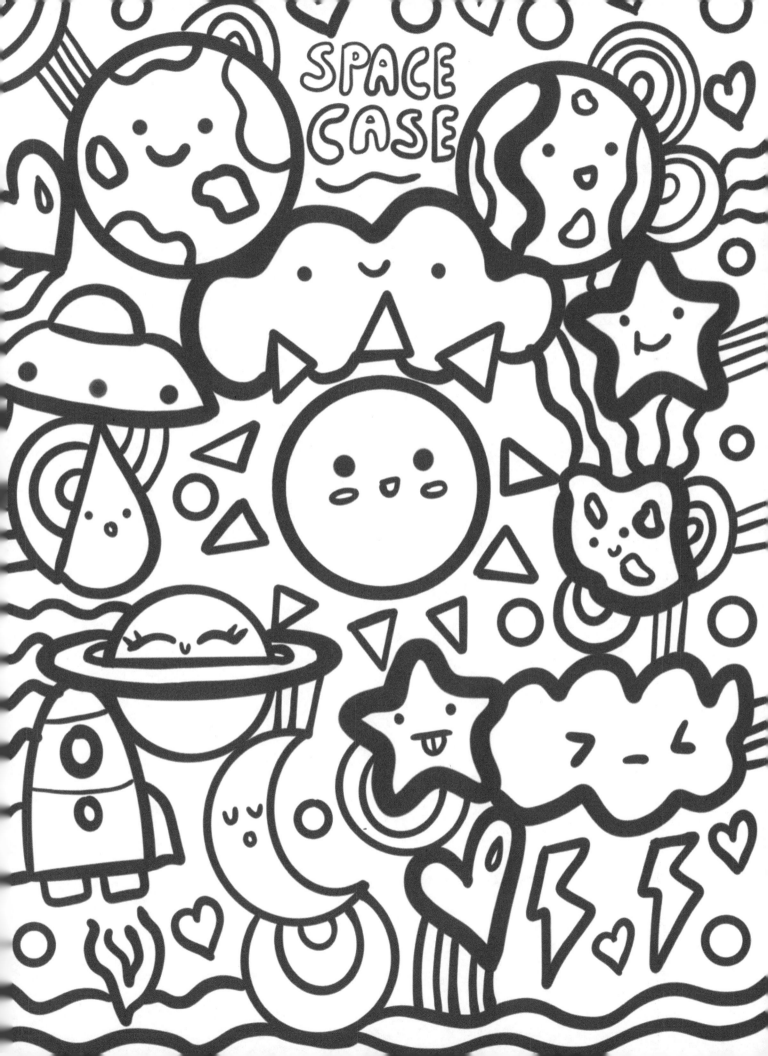

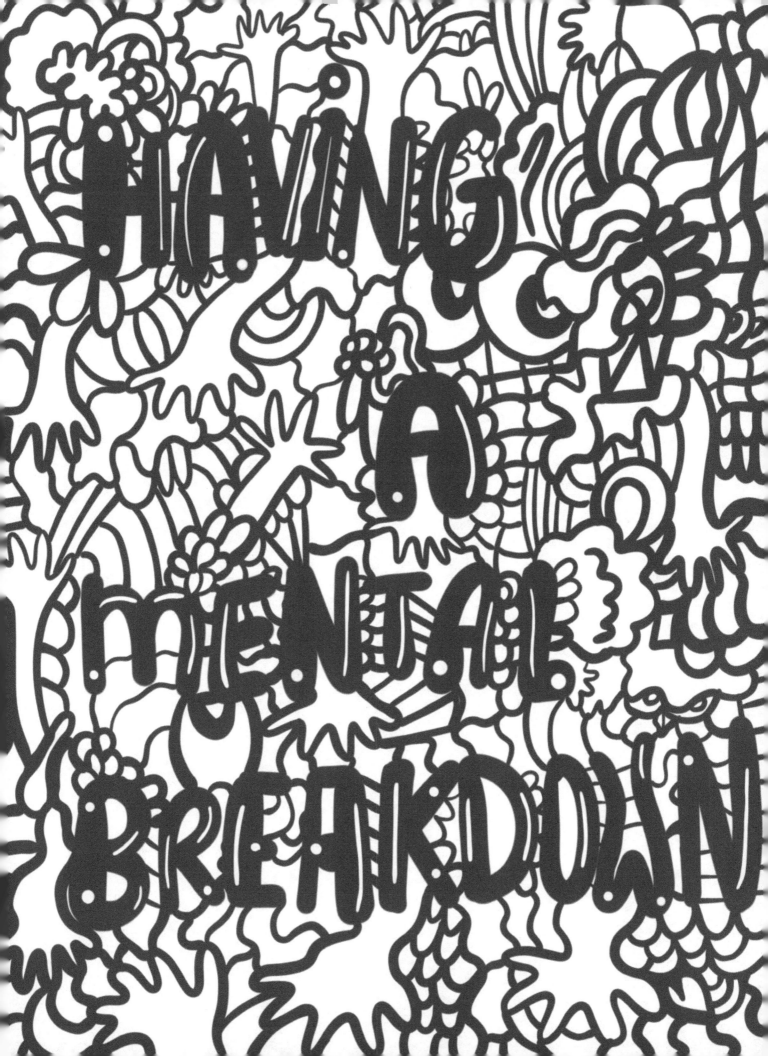

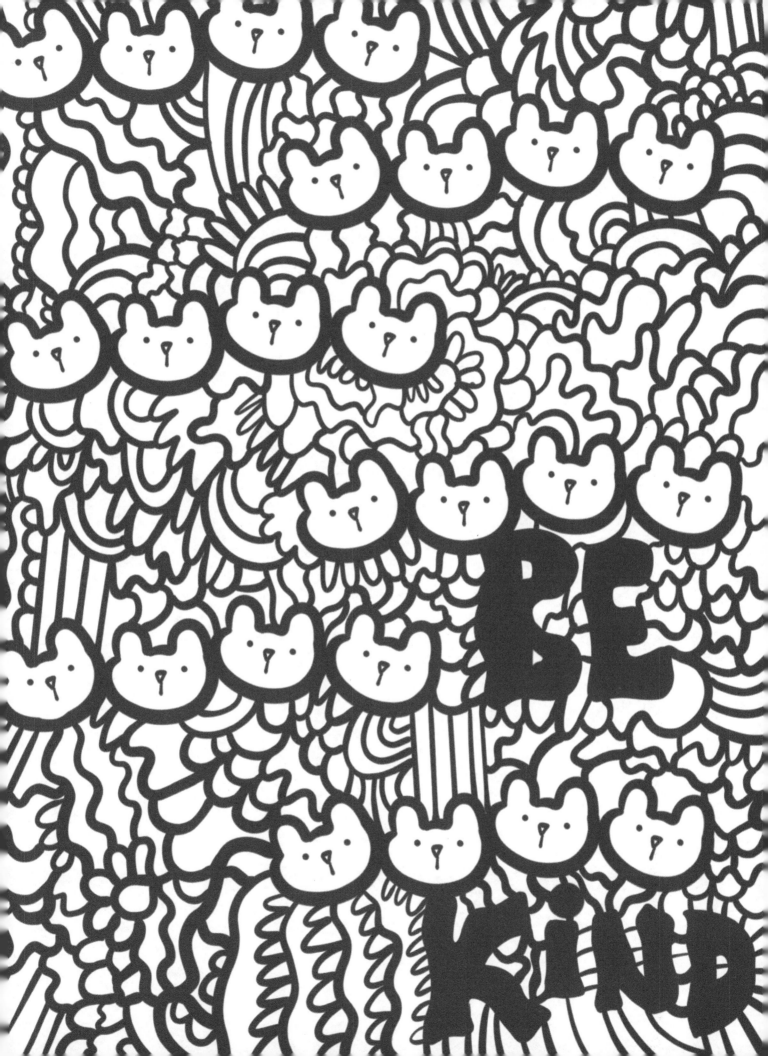

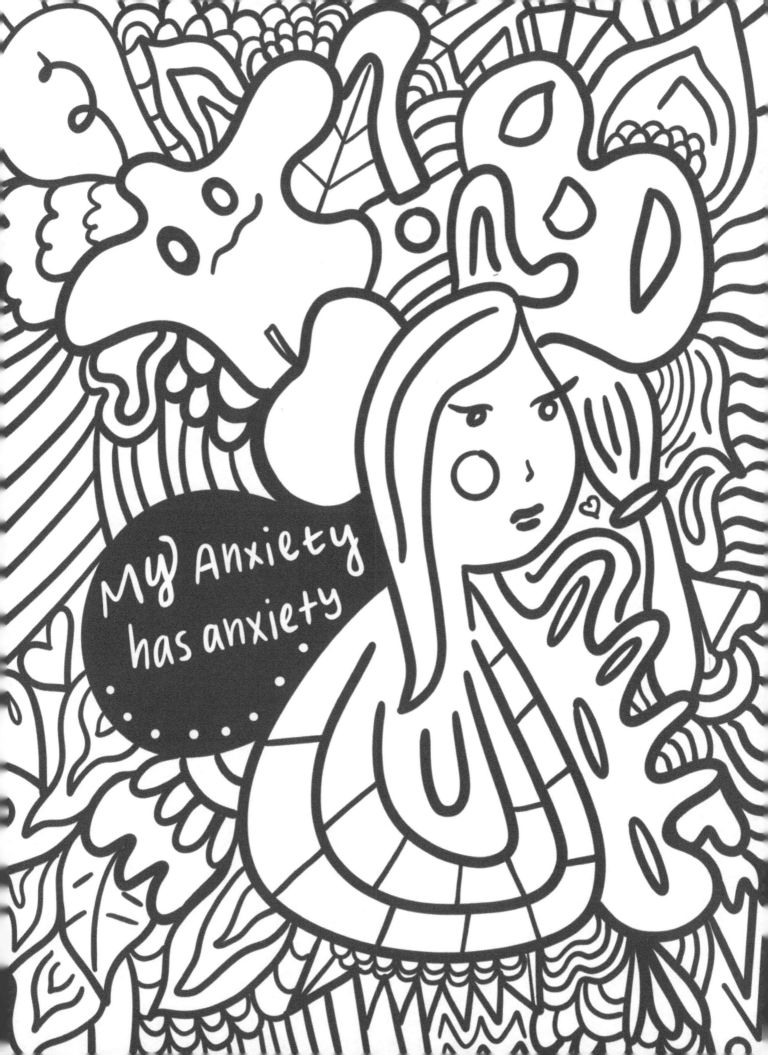

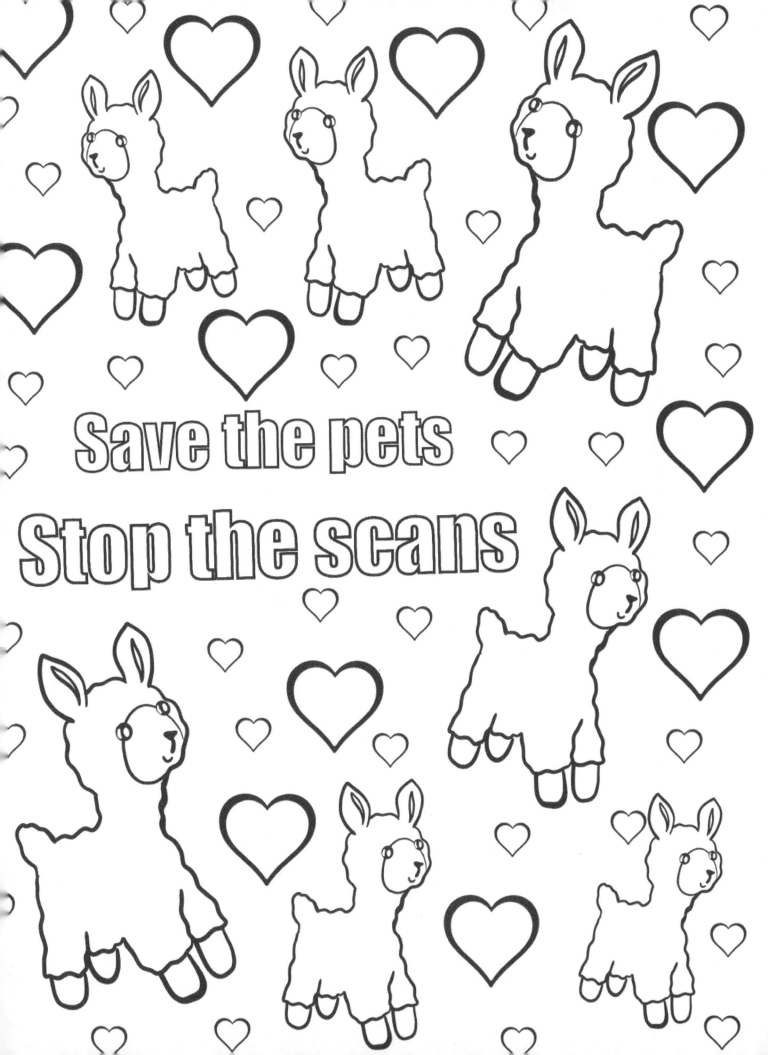

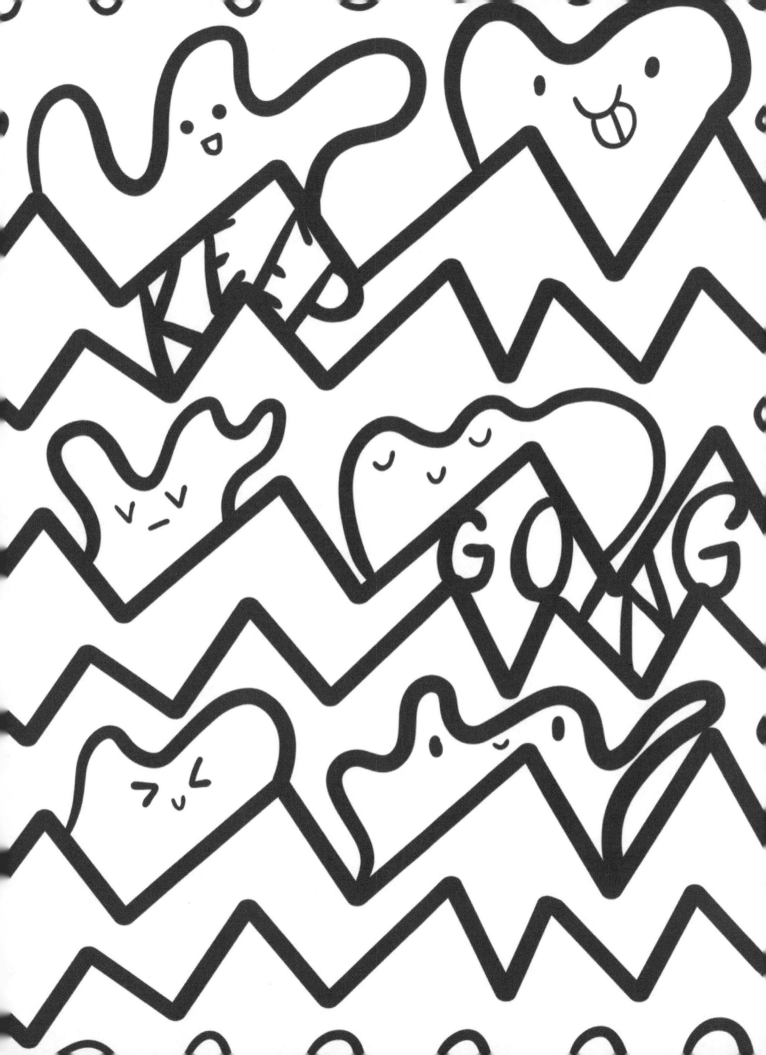

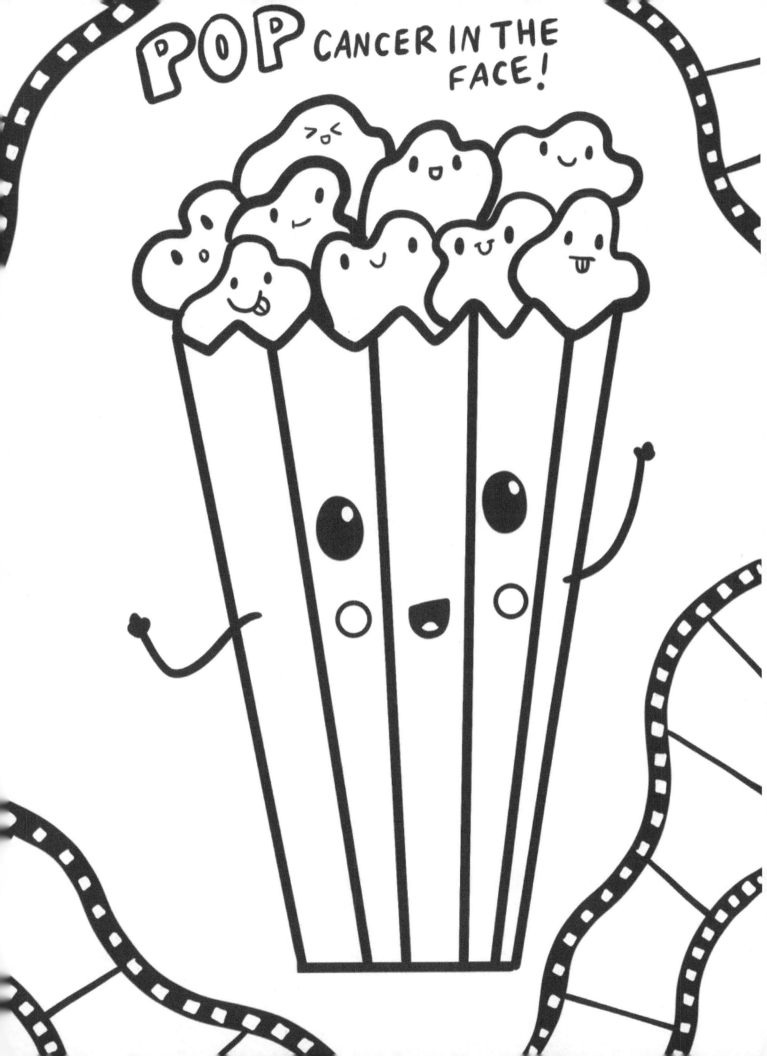

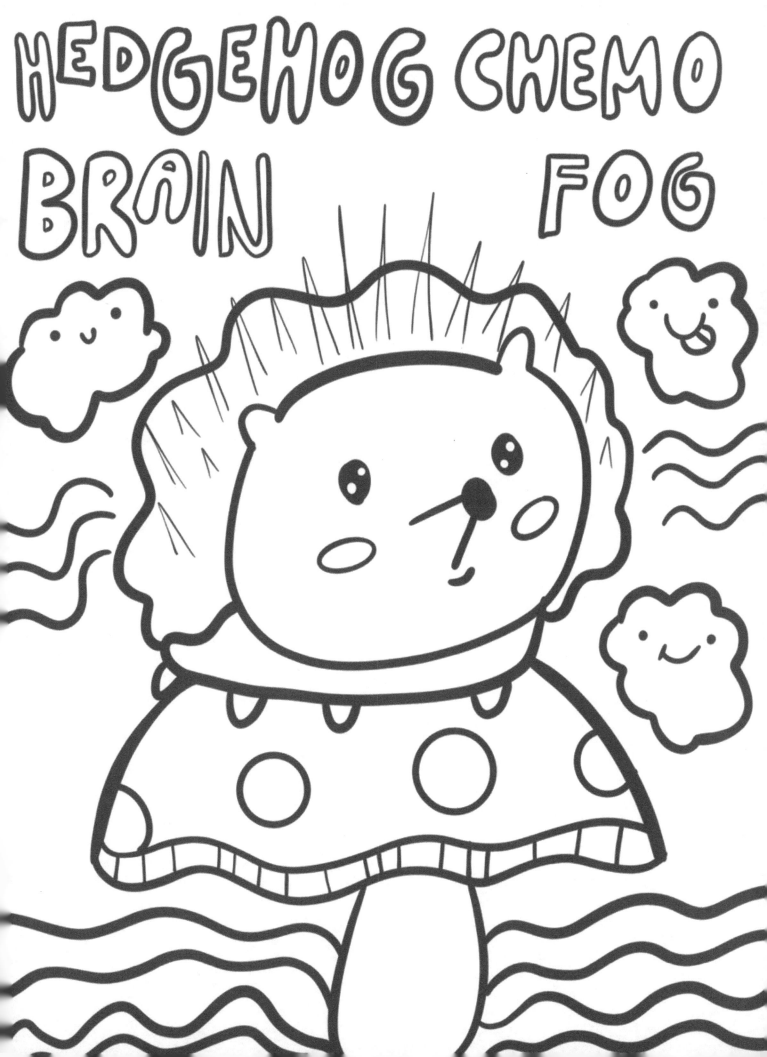

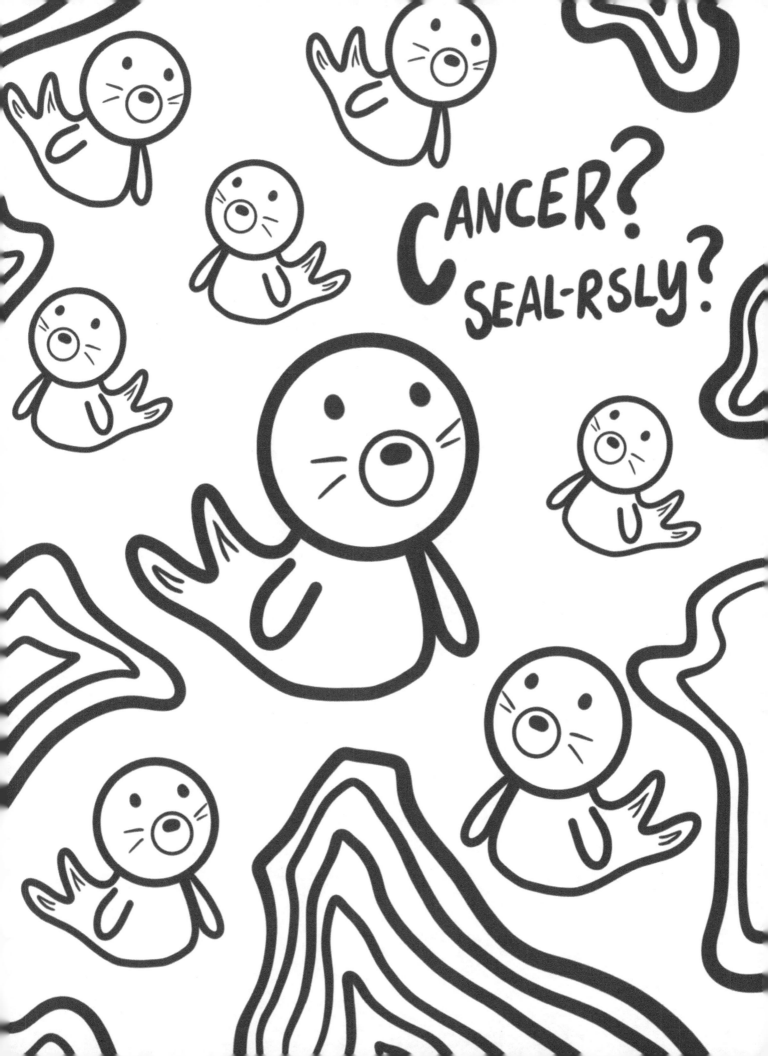

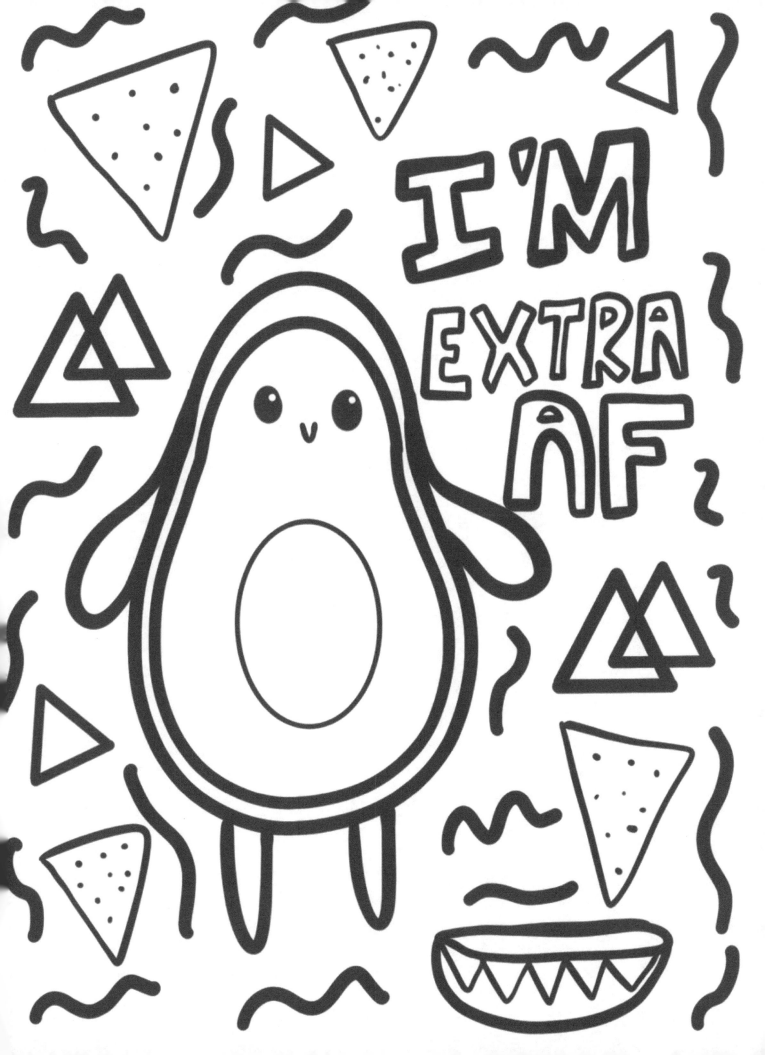

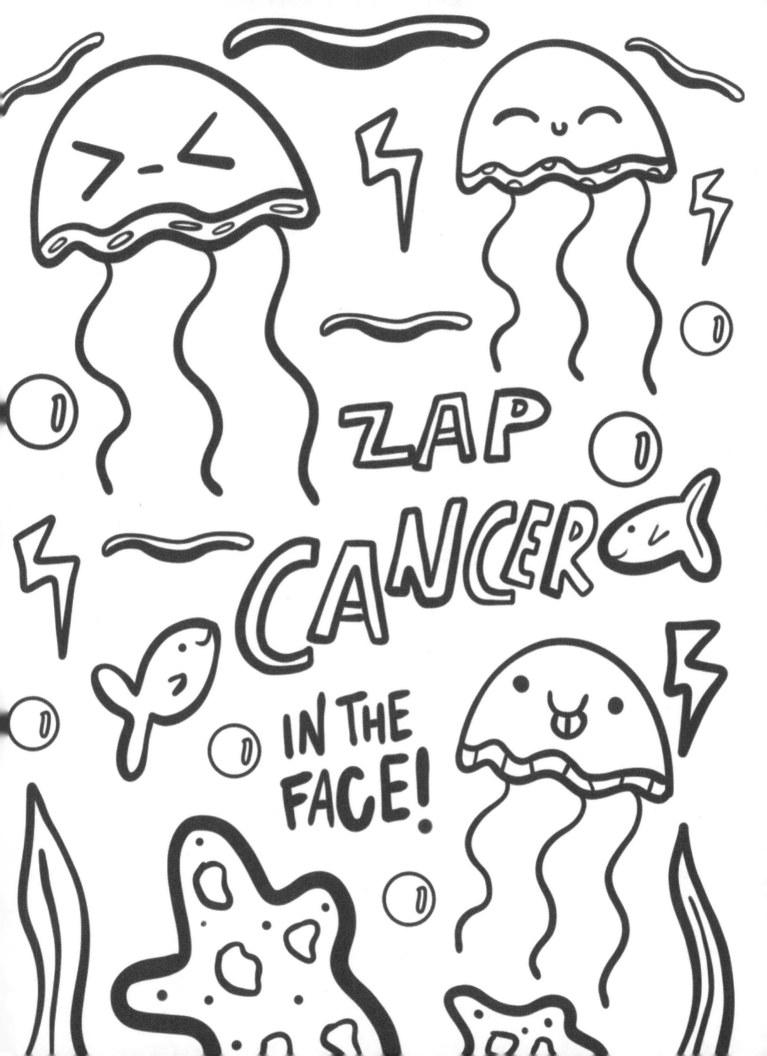

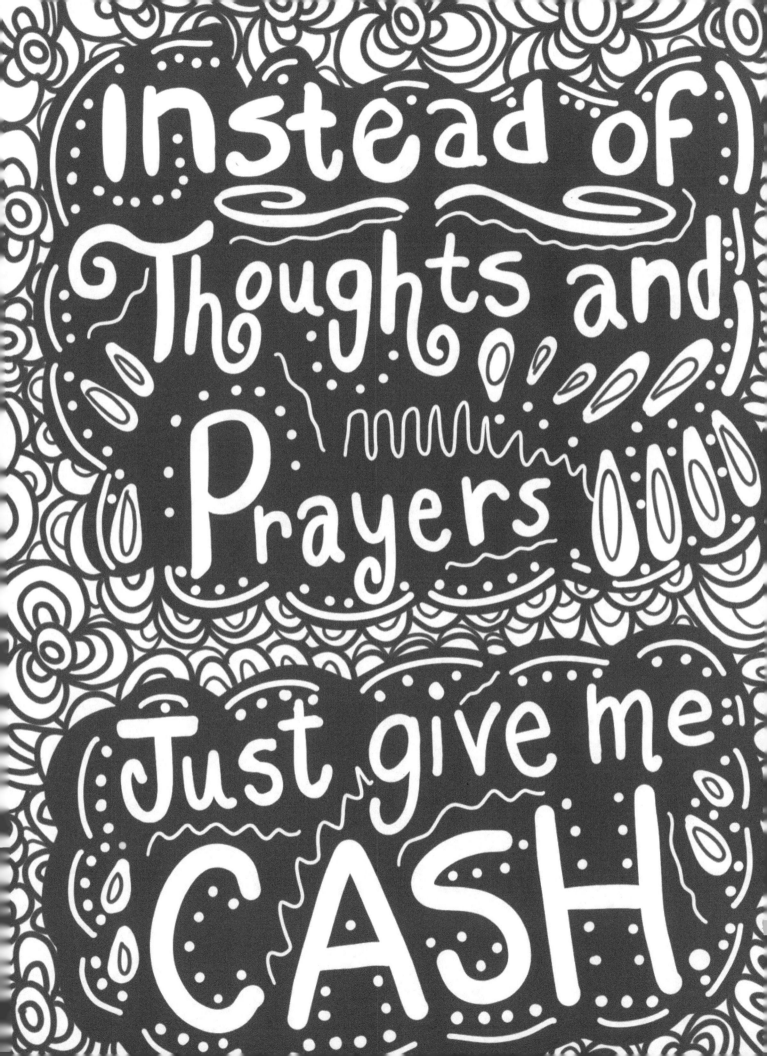

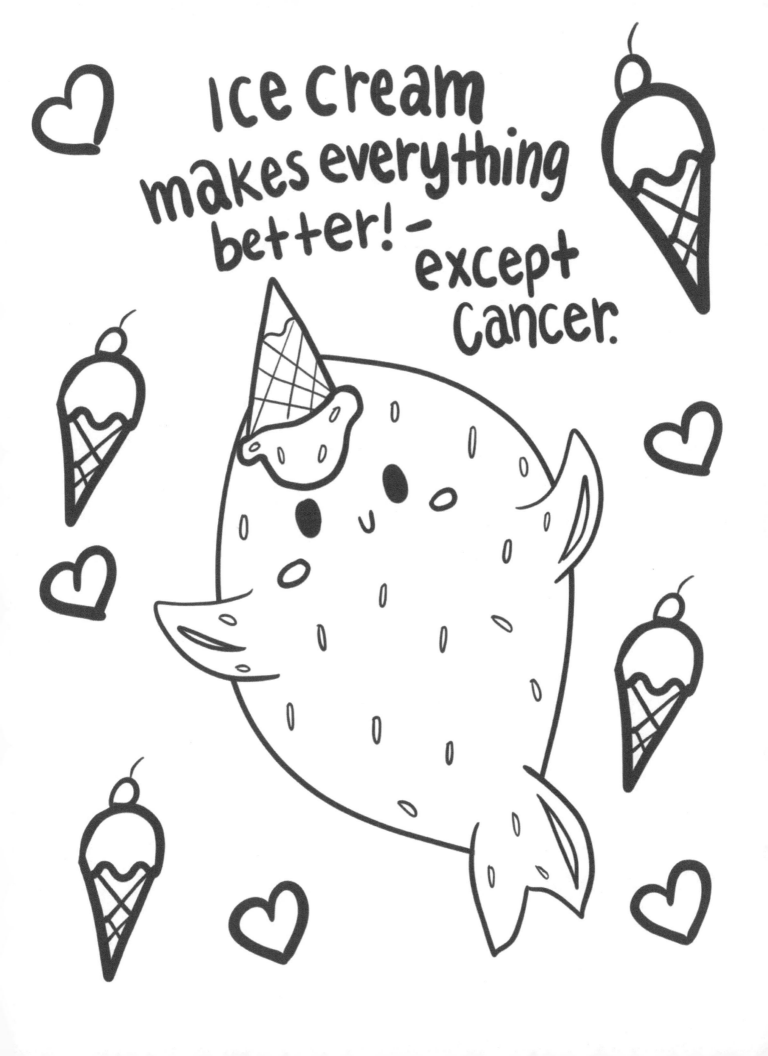

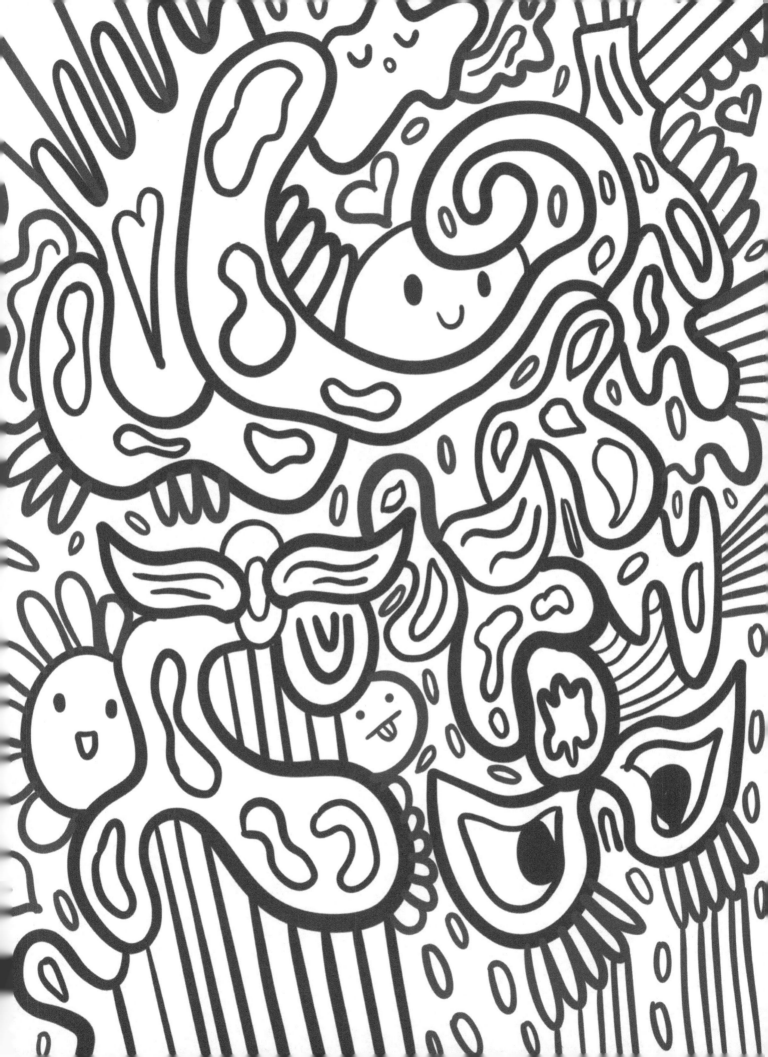

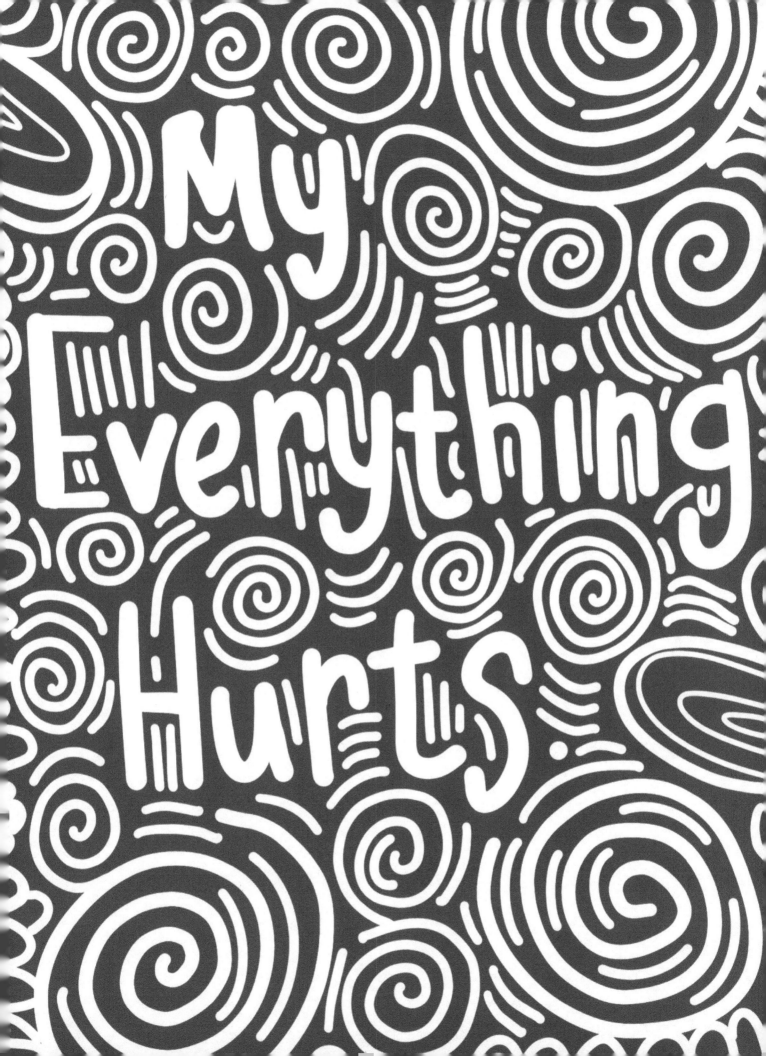

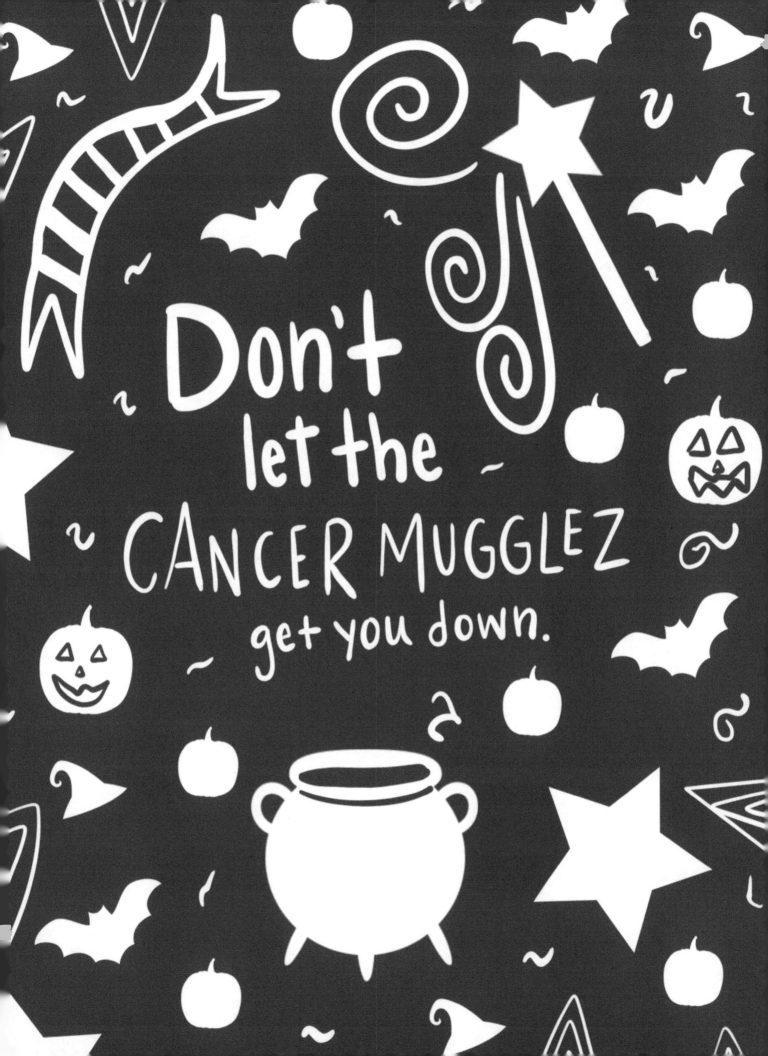

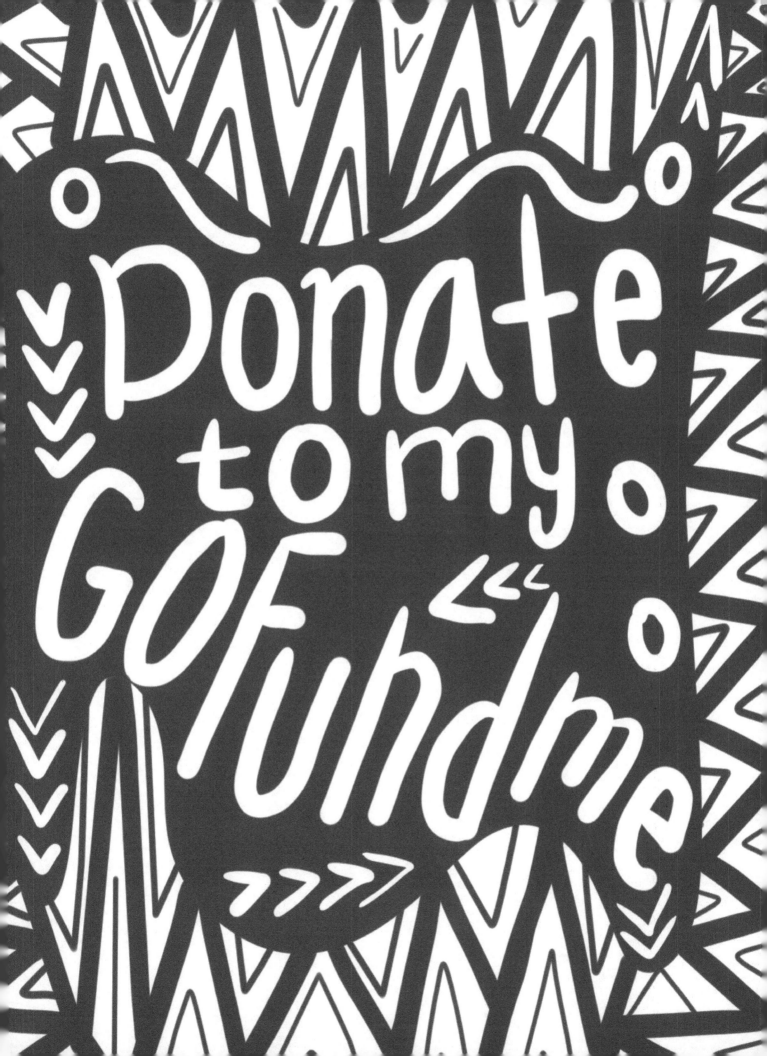

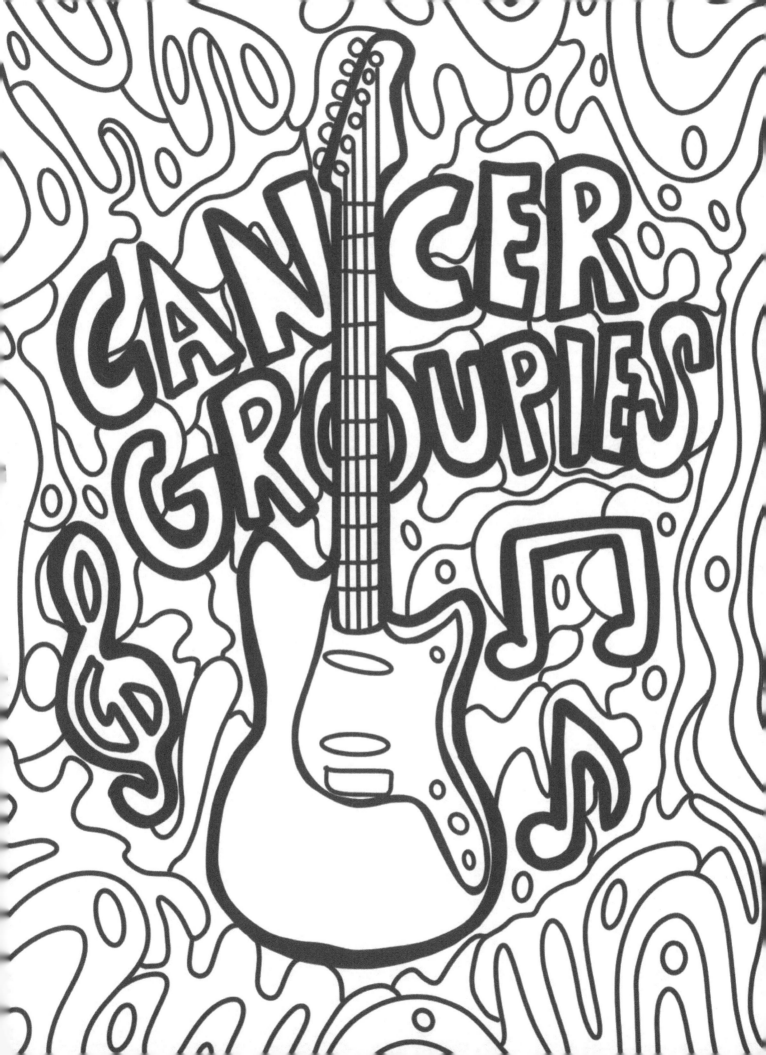

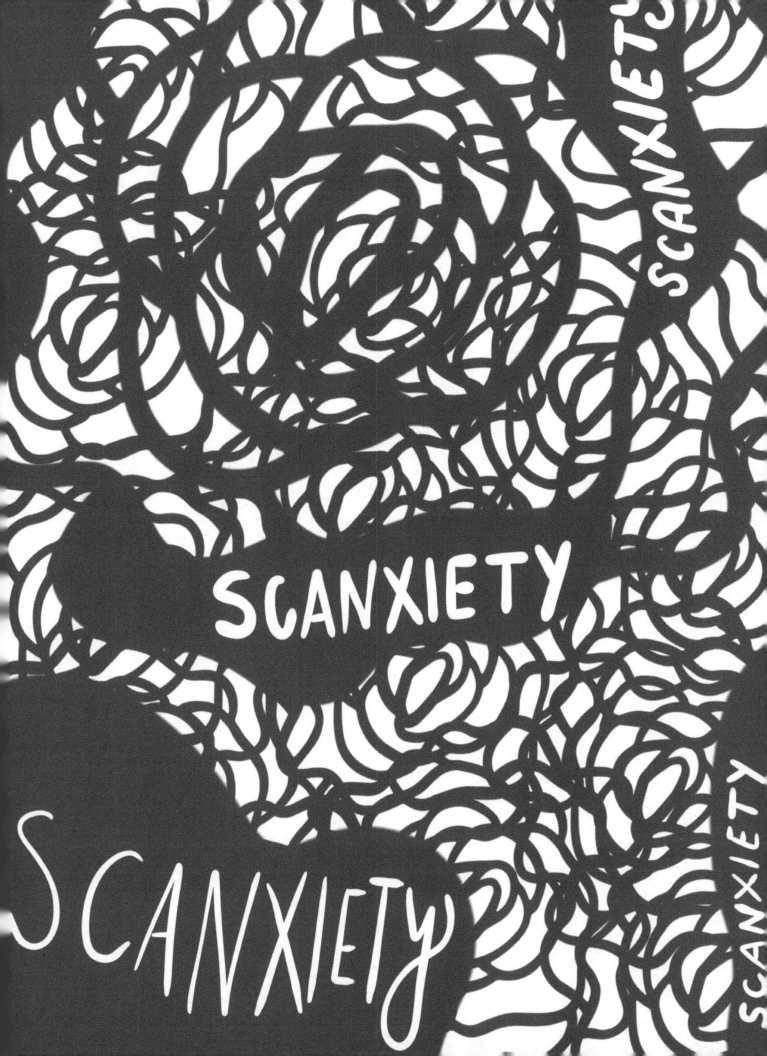

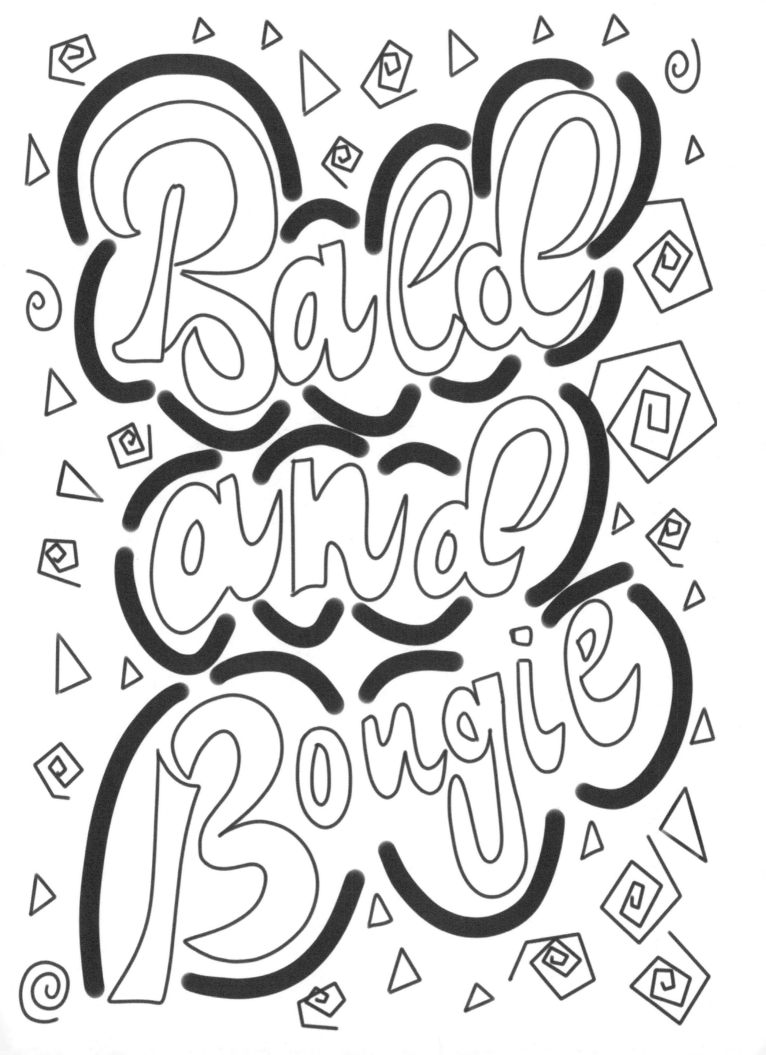

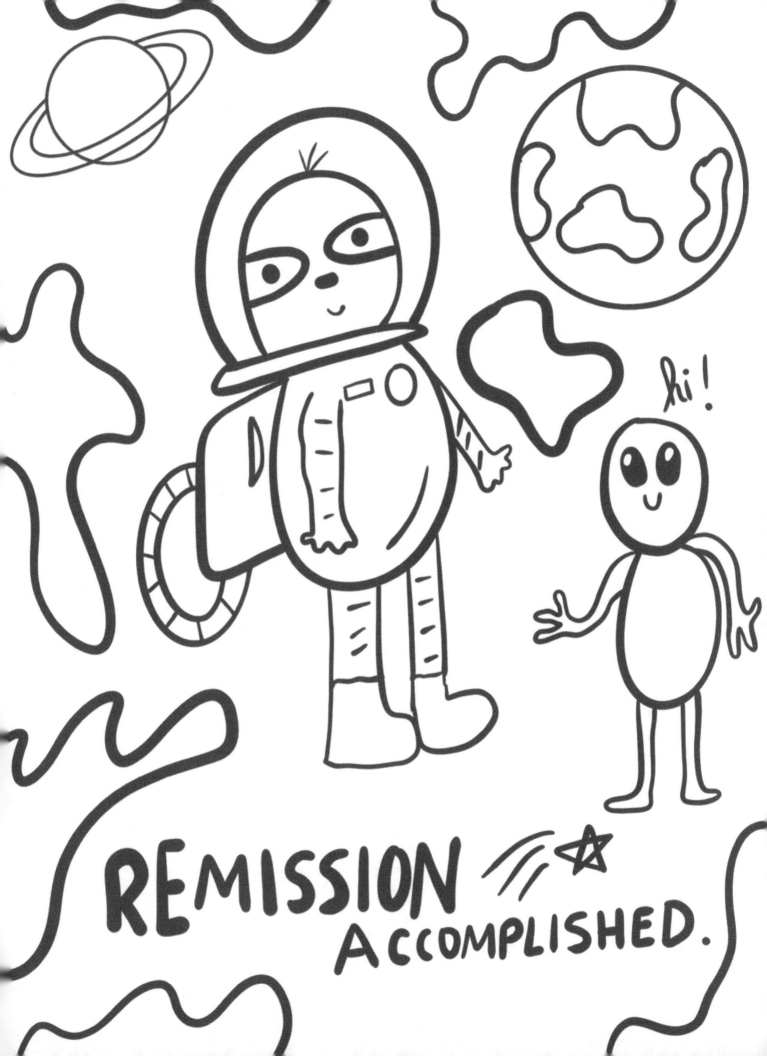

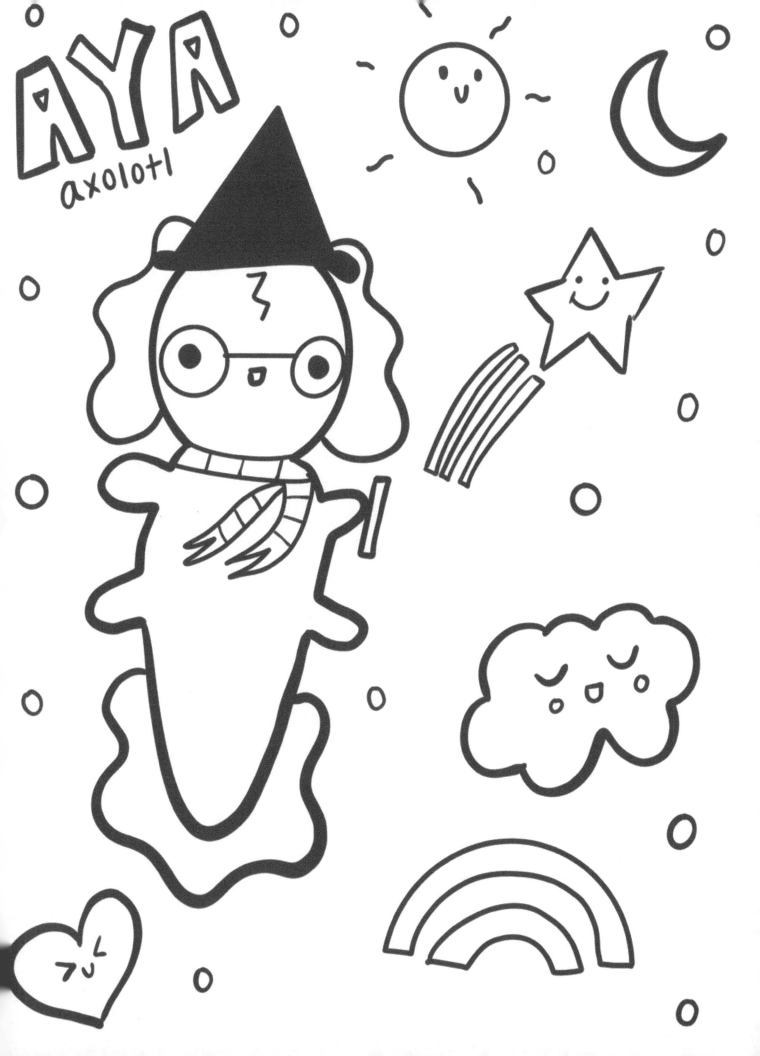

AYA
axolotl

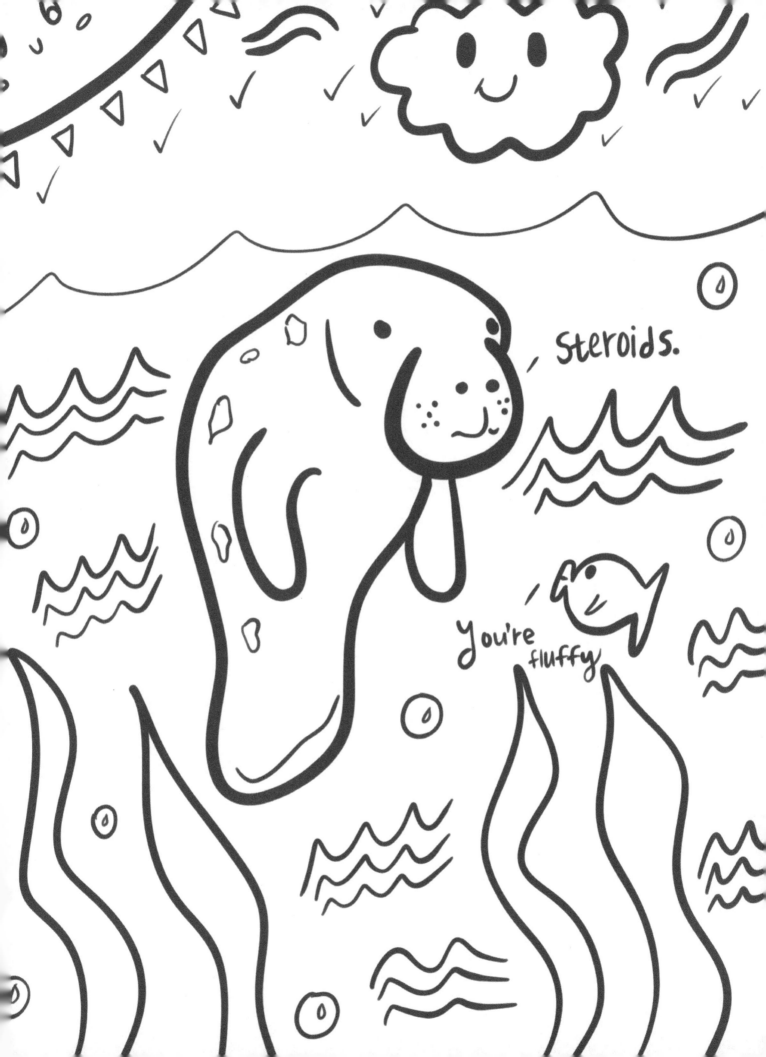

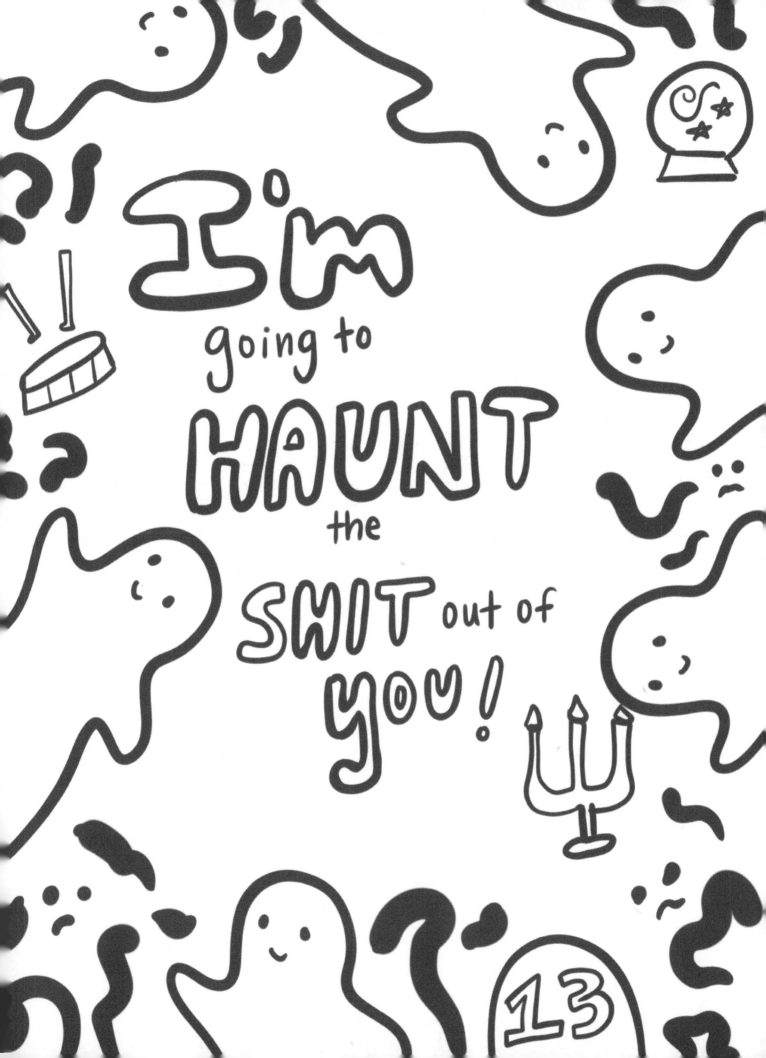

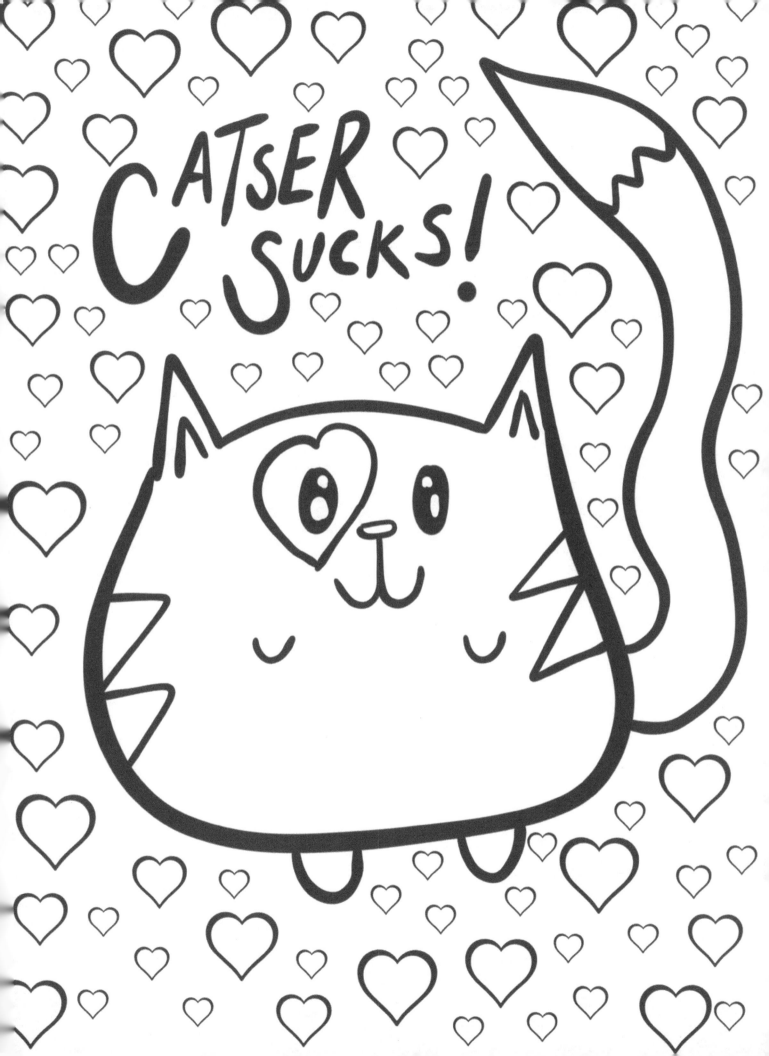

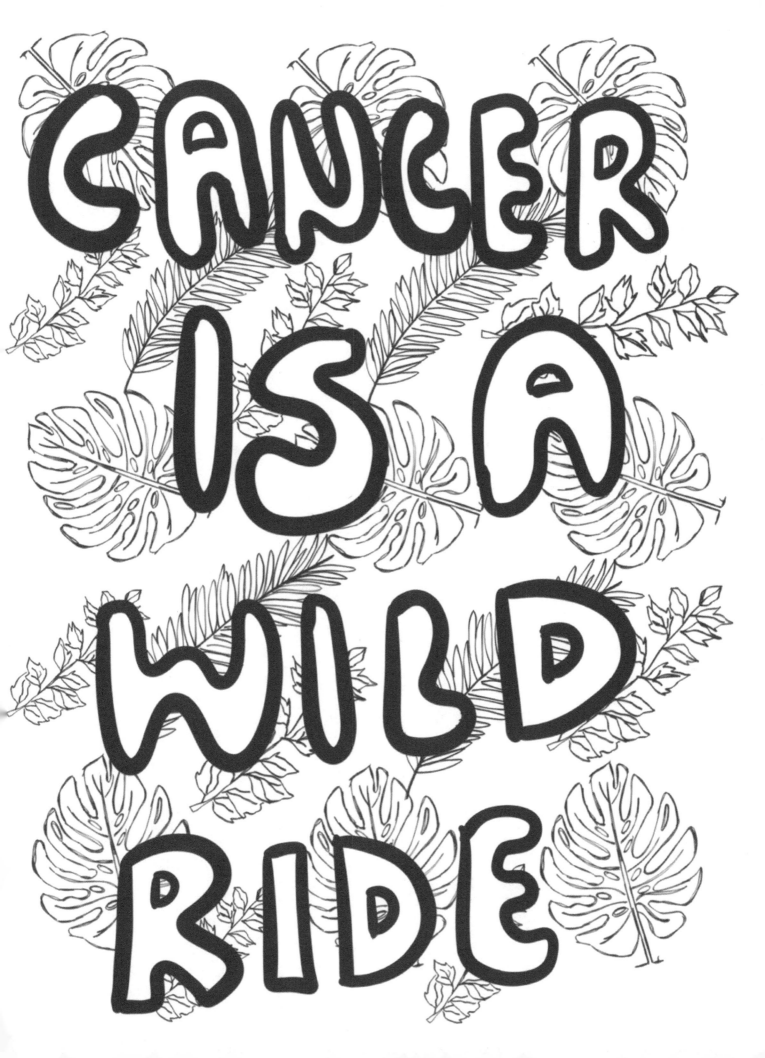

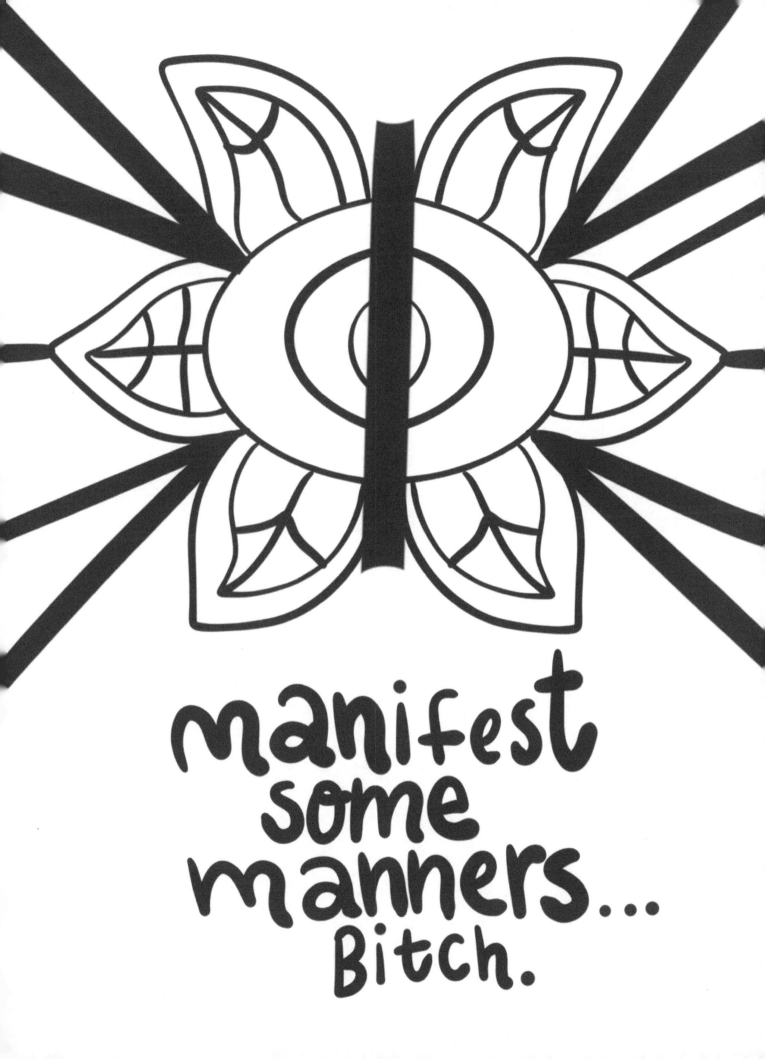

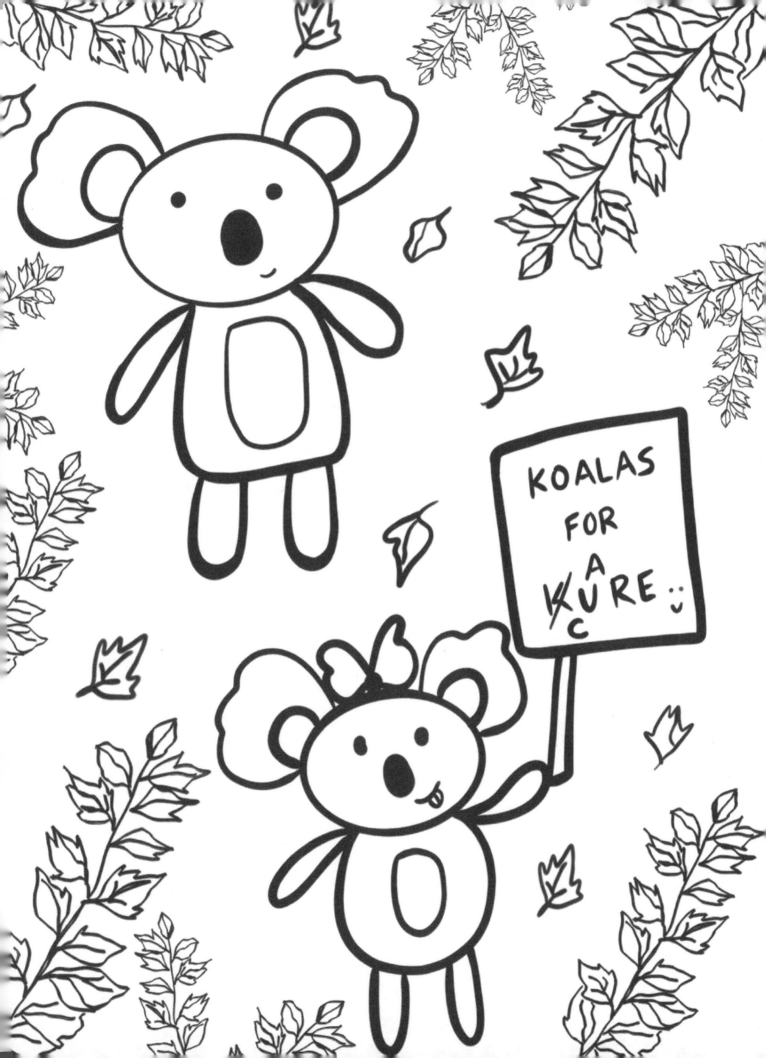

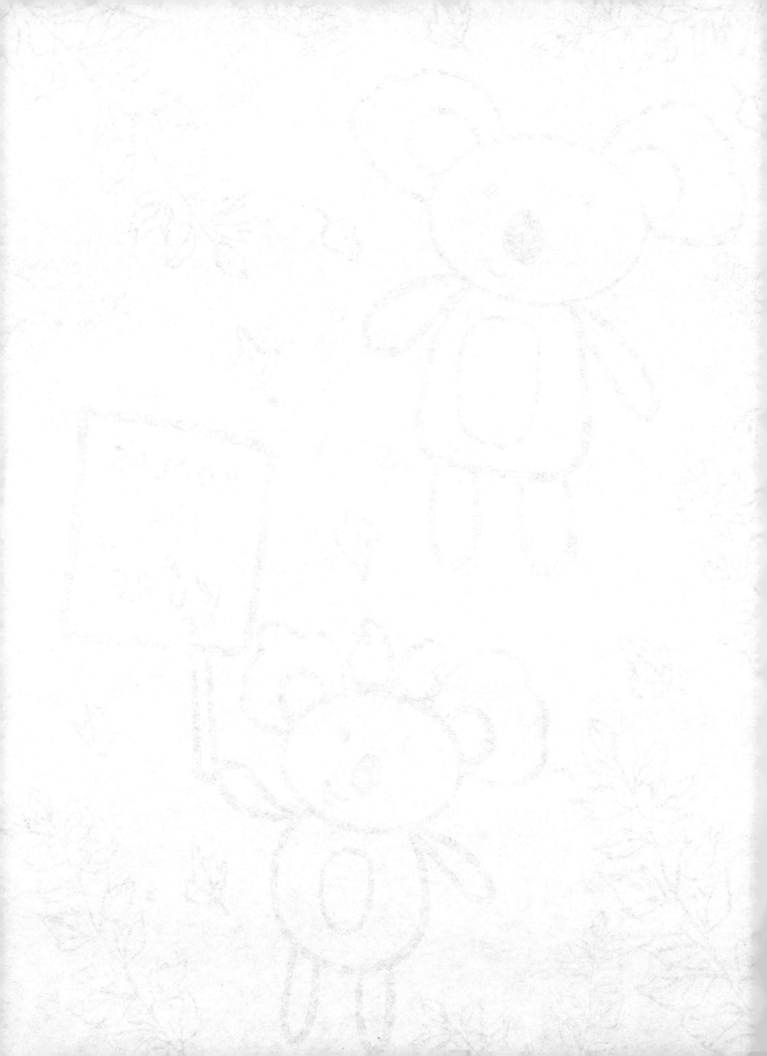

Made in United States
Cleveland, OH
27 July 2025

18883749R00050